EAT HEALTHY

LIVE HEALTHY

WHAT AND HOW TO EAT TO STAY HEALTHY, IN SHAPE AND STRONG

BY

DR. DONALD CLINTON

Contents

Introduction

Starting an eating routine to shed pounds and further develop wellbeing is a commendable objective, however it tends to a piece overpower. There will undoubtedly be difficulties at whatever point you begin a novel, new thing, particularly when it includes something you complete a few times every day - - like eating and drinking.

In any case, as long as you don't attempt to change everything simultaneously, you can meet your weight reduction objectives. Peruse on to gain proficiency with certain mysteries of the bosses - - the individuals who have shed pounds and, all the more significantly, kept it off. All things considered, what benefit is losing the additional weight on the off chance that you gain it right

back?

Chapter One

Ways to Get Your Diet off to a Good Start

1. Follow a Healthy Eating Plan

A good dieting plan (like the WebMD Weight Loss Clinic plan) ought to incorporate food varieties you appreciate alongside a lot of solid, not-too-handled food sources like natural products, vegetables, entire grains, low-fat dairy, lean meats, fish, beans, and nuts. On account of their capacity to fulfill, these low-calorie food varieties will really assist you with adhering to your eating routine. The most fulfilling food sources have loads of fiber (like natural products, vegetables, entire grains, beans, and nuts) and additionally low-fat protein (tracked down in meat, fish, dairy, and soy).

In a perfect world, you'll gradually wean yourself off most loved food sources that are vigorously handled and high in fat or calories, and supplant them with additional nutritious choices. Whenever during this cycle, go ahead and think of another eating plan that cxpands a few invigorating food sources and diminishes others. It's best for WLC individuals to make another arrangement toward the week's end. At the point when you do as such, the WLC electronic diary starts all over again

You can definitely relax in the event that you are a vegan, or have sensitivities or bigotries. Your customized WLC eating plan may exclude all of the suggested nutrition types, yet it will give satisfactory supplements.

We suggest that everybody take an everyday multivitamin/mineral enhancement to fill in any dietary holes.

Change is hard. Making little, steady changes in your eating designs is the most ideal way to upgrade your eating routine. A few specialists propose rolling out only one improvement every week, to give you an opportunity to become acclimated to the new way of behaving. Your definitive objective is to lay out new dietary patterns that can be supported for a lifetime.

You can loosen up if you are a veggie lover, or have responsive qualities or bigotries. Your altered WLC eating plan might reject all of the recommended nourishment types, yet it will give acceptable enhancements. We recommend that everyone take a regular multivitamin/mineral upgrade to fill in any dietary openings.

2. Take Baby Steps

Change is hard. Making nearly nothing, consistent changes in your eating plans is the best method for updating your eating schedule. A couple of experts propose carrying out just a single improvement consistently, to offer you a chance to become adjusted to the better approach for acting. Your conclusive goal is to spread out new dietary examples that can be upheld for a lifetime.

3. Put forth Realistic Goals

The vast majority who need to get more fit put forth grandiose objectives, longing for squeezing into dress sizes that may not be sensible for them. However losing just 5% to 10% of your body weight can further develop the manner in which you feel, put a flash in your step, and, in particular, work on your wellbeing. Concentrates on show that terrible even limited quantities of weight can work on generally speaking wellbeing and, explicitly, lower circulatory strain, and glucose and cholesterol levels.

Put forth weight reduction objectives that are feasible, and remember that the suggested pace of weight reduction is just 1-2 pounds each week. Gradual comes out on top in this race. It requires investment to learn new dietary patterns that will keep going until the end of your life.

4. Reward, Don't Punish

To keep inspiration high, reward yourself in the wake of coming to mini goals. All things considered, shedding 5 pounds or coming to the exercise center multiple times in seven days merits a gesture of congratulations.

Then again, don't be too unforgiving with yourself when you tumble off the cart - - everybody does, sometime. Guess that slipups will occur, and when they do, simply get over yourself and get right in the groove again. Utilize your slipup to realize where you are helpless, and conclude how you will deal with the circumstance the following time without leaving your eating regimen. My idea is attempt to do your best 80% of the time, and loosen up the principles to some degree the other 20% of the time.

5. Get a Buddy

Support is a fundamental piece of a fruitful get-healthy plan. Enroll a relative, track down a companion to go along with you in your strolls or exercises, and engage in the WLC online local area. These individuals will turn into a wellspring of motivation, backing, and consolation consistently - - and particularly whenever difficult situations arise.

6. Track Your Meals

Fruitful washouts know that it is so essential to record what and the amount they eat. The basic demonstration of recording a useful asset can assist with keeping you in charge.

Utilize the WLC diary capability, or on the other hand assuming you like, keep your own journal to follow your day to day food admission.

7. Add Exercise

Eating restoratively and cutting calories is just around 50% of the equation for fruitful weight reduction. Getting customary actual work is the other piece. Practice is an integral asset, assisting you with consuming calories and increment strength, equilibrium, and coordination while diminishing pressure and working on your general wellbeing.

My recommendation is to fit in wellness first thing, to ensure it doesn't get extracted from your bustling day. (Prior to beginning any work out regime, check with your primary care physician, and keeping in mind that you're busy, bring your PCP a duplicate of your eating intend to examine.)

You ought to be pleased that you have gone with the choice to work on your wellbeing. Realize that the street ahead will have a few knocks, yet furnished with a decent eating plan, emotionally supportive network, and an uplifting perspective, you will find success. Best of luck

14

Chapter Two

Common Reasons Why You're Not Losing as Much Weight as You Expected To

At the point when you get thinner, your body retaliates. You might have the option to lose a considerable amount of weight from the outset, absent a lot of exertion. Notwithstanding, weight reduction might dial back or stop out and out sooner or later.

This chapter records 15 normal motivations behind for what reason you're not getting in shape.

It additionally contains noteworthy hints on the most proficient method to get through the level and get things rolling once more.

1. Perhaps You Are Losing Without Acknowledging It

On the off chance that you assume you are encountering a weight reduction level, you shouldn't worry at this time. It is unimaginably normal for the scale not to move for a couple of days (or weeks) at a time. This doesn't imply that you are not losing fat.

Body weight will in general vary by a couple of pounds. It relies upon the food varieties you are eating, and chemicals can likewise significantly affect how much water your body holds (particularly in ladies).

Likewise, it is feasible to acquire muscle simultaneously as you lose fat. This is especially normal assuming that you as of late begun working out. This is something worth being thankful for, as what you truly need to lose is muscle versus fat, not simply weight. It is really smart to utilize some different option from the scale to measure your advancement. For instance, measure your midsection boundary and muscle versus fat ratio one time each month.

Likewise, how well your garments fit and how you search in the mirror can very tell. Except if your weight has been stuck at similar point for more than 1 fourteen days, you likely don't have to stress over anything.

2. You're not Monitoring What You're Eating

Mindfulness is extraordinarily significant in the event that you are attempting to get in shape. Many individuals haven't the foggiest idea the amount they're truly eating. Concentrates on show that monitoring your food admission assists with weight reduction. Individuals who use food journals or photo their dinners reliably lose more weight than individuals who don't.

Simultaneously, there is an expected drawback to food following, particularly when it's utilized with the end goal of weight reduction.

3. You're Not Eating Sufficient Protein

Protein is a significant supplement for getting thinner. Eating protein at 25-30% of calories can help digestion by 80-100 calories each day and make you naturally eat a few hundred less calories each day. It can likewise definitely diminish desires and craving for nibbling

Assuming you have breakfast, make certain to stack up on protein. Concentrates on show that the people who have a high protein breakfast are less eager and have less desires over the course of the day. A high protein consumption likewise forestalls metabolic lull, a typical symptom of getting more fit. Furthermore, it forestalls weight recover.

4. You're Eating an Excessive Number of Calories

Many individuals who experience difficulty getting thinner are essentially eating such a large number of calories.

You might imagine that this doesn't concern you, however remember that concentrates reliably show that individuals will generally misjudge their calorie consumption overwhelmingly.

On the off chance that you are not getting more fit, you ought to take a stab at gauging your food varieties and following your calories for some time.

Here are a few supportive assets:

Calorie adding machine. Utilize a calorie mini-computer to sort out the number of calories to eat.

Calorie counters. This is a rundown of five free sites and applications that can assist you with monitoring your calorie and supplement consumption.

Following is likewise significant in the event that you're attempting to arrive at a specific supplement objective, for example, getting 30% of your calories from protein.

This can be difficult to accomplish in the event that you're not following things appropriately.

It is by and large not important to count calories and weigh everything until the end of your life. All things considered, evaluate these methods for a couple of days like clockwork to discover the amount you're eating.

5. You're Not Eating Entire Food Sources

Food quality is similarly just about as significant as amount.

Eating entire food varieties can further develop your prosperity and assist with directing your craving. These food varieties will generally be substantially more filling than their exceptionally handled partners.

Remember that many handled food sources marked as "wellbeing food varieties" aren't exactly solid. Make certain to peruse the fixings on the bundle and watch out for food varieties containing extra crabs.

6. You're Not Lifting Loads

Perhaps of the main thing you can do while getting in shape is to do some type of obstruction preparing, for example, lifting loads.

This can assist you with keeping up with bulk, which is frequently singed alongside muscle to fat ratio in the event that you are not working out.

Lifting loads can likewise assist with forestalling metabolic lull and guarantee that your body stays conditioned and strong.

7. You're Voraciously Consuming Food

Gorging includes quickly eating a lot of food, frequently considerably more than your body needs.

This can be a huge issue for some individuals attempting to get thinner. Some might gorge on profoundly handled food sources, while others gorge on generally good food varieties, including nuts, nut spreads, dull chocolate, cheddar, and so forth. Regardless of whether something is considered "sound," its calories actually count.

8. You're not Hitting the Treadmill

Cardiovascular activity, otherwise called cardio or high-impact work out, is any kind of activity that expands your pulse. It incorporates exercises like running, cycling, and swimming.

It is one of the best ways of working on your wellbeing.

It is likewise exceptionally powerful at consuming paunch fat, the hurtful instinctive fat that develops around your organs and causes illness.

9. You're Actually Drinking Sugar

Sweet drinks are essentially swelling things in the food supply. Your mind doesn't make up for the calories in them by causing you to eat less of different food varieties.

This isn't just valid for sweet beverages like Coke and Pepsi. It additionally applies to "better" drinks like Vitamin water, which are additionally stacked with sugar.

Indeed, even organic product juices are tricky and ought not to be polished off in enormous sums. A solitary glass can contain a comparative measure of sugar as a few bits of entire natural product.

10. You're not Resting Soundly

Great rest is one of the main variables for your physical and emotional wellness as well as your weight.

Concentrates on show that unfortunate rest is one of the single greatest gamble factors for heftiness. Grown-ups and kids with unfortunate rest have a 55% and 89% more serious gamble, individually, for creating weight.

11. You're Not Scaling Back Sugars

In the event that you have a higher measure of weight to lose as well as you have a metabolic condition like sort 2 diabetes or pre-diabetes, you might need to consider a low crab diet.

In transient examinations, this sort of diet has been displayed to cause up to 2-3 fold the amount of weight reduction as the norm "low fat" diet that is frequently suggested.

Then again, a later preliminary in 2018 found little contrast in the consequences of a supplement thick, low fat eating regimen versus a supplement thick, low carb diet. Finding a reasonable dinner plan that you can appreciate long haul is critical.

Low crab eats less crabs have numerous up-sides past weight reduction. They can likewise prompt upgrades in numerous metabolic markers, like fatty oils, HDL (great) cholesterol, and glucose.

12. You're Eating Time And Again

It is a fantasy that everybody ought to eat numerous little dinners every day to help digestion and get in shape.

It is additionally ludicrously awkward to plan and eating food the entire day, as it makes solid nourishment considerably more confounded.

Then again, one powerful weight reduction strategy called discontinuous fasting includes purposely and decisively doing without nourishment for broadened timeframes (15-24 hours or more).

13. You're Not Drinking Water

Drinking water can help weight reduction.

In one 12-week weight reduction study, individuals who drank a portion of a liter (17 ounces) of water 30 minutes before feasts lost 44% more weight than the people who didn't.

Drinking water has likewise been displayed to help the quantity of calories consumed by 24-30% over a time of 90 minutes.

14. You're Drinking an Excessive Amount Of Liquor

If you like liquor however need to get thinner, it very well might be ideal to adhere to spirits (like vodka) blended in with a zero-calorie refreshment. Brew, wine, and sweet cocktails are extremely high in calories.

Additionally remember that the actual liquor has around 7 calories for each gram, which is high.

That being expressed, concentrates on liquor and weight show blended results. Moderate drinking is by all accounts fine, while weighty drinking is connected to weight gain.

15. You're not Eating Carefully

A procedure called careful eating might be one of the world's most impressive weight reduction devices.

It includes dialing back, eating without interruption, relishing and partaking in each nibble while paying attention to the regular signals that let your mind know when your body has had enough.

Various investigations have demonstrated the way that careful eating can cause huge weight reduction and decrease the recurrence of voraciously consuming food.

Chapter Three

Simple Ways to Burn Fat without Losing Muscle

The capacity for you to consume fat and construct muscle reduces to your eating routine and exercise propensities. There are a lot of wellness devotees who've achieved these objectives all the while, filling in as episodic proof that accomplishing body decomposition is conceivable. Follow these hints to consume fat without losing hard-acquired muscle.

1. Consolidate Strength With Hypertrophy

Unadulterated strength preparing, like lifting weighty singles, pairs, or triples, depends vigorously on your brain drive, the speed you shift from utilizing Type I to

Type II muscle filaments, and your capacity to get maximal muscle fiber enlistment. While those are very helpful for setting PR's in the center, they don't expand how much muscle you put on or keep up with during a cutting stage.

All things considered, join both to make an extraordinary muscle-building exercise. For instance, do five weighty reps, rest for 20 seconds, rehash that equivalent definite load for three reps, rest for 20 seconds, and afterward do two additional reps. You're as yet ready to utilize an exceptionally significant burden, however you made it keep going for 10 reps. This makes an enormous improvement for thicker muscles and the "siphon".

2.   Utilize Slow Aerobic Cardio

With fat misfortune comes cardio preparing. However the sort of cardio you really do can keep up with all your well deserved muscle or annihilate it.

Utilize slow and simple strategies for oxygen consuming activity, for example, strolling on a treadmill at a grade, a simple bicycle ride, or a light run. Keeping a simple speed will just utilize your Type I muscle strands, which are very exhaustion safe, and elevate more blood course to assist with clearing lactic corrosive and metabolic waste. It additionally further develops your vigorous energy framework to help more serious exercises, better recuperation among sets, and more outcomes.

3.   Eat More Lean Protein

To keep up with however much as could be expected (on the off chance that not, develop it) during a cutting stage, you consume the ideal measure of protein. In the first place, it helps your digestion over the course of the day since protein takes more energy to process than crabs or fat. Second, it keeps you full to forestall gorging.

At last, it forestalls unnecessary muscle misfortune that could occur during a cut. Focus no less than 1g of protein per pound of bodyweight, and get your protein from clean sources like lean meats, nuts, eggs, fish, and quality enhancements.

4.   Rest 8 Hours per Night

Recuperation is similarly pretty much as significant as your preparation, particularly during a cutting stage. Since you're putting your body through the huge pressure of calorie-limitation and significant burdens, you want time to allow your muscles to recuperate and modify.

While your body secretes development chemical over the course of the day, it tops around evening time while you rest and it's likewise most elevated when your rest is most profound. Holding back on rest, be that as it may, will just bamboozle your muscle development and fix.

5.   Keep up with Only a Moderate Caloric Deficit

Crash diets will cause muscle misfortune regardless of what you do. It's very outrageous on the body and won't give your body an adequate number of supplements to recuperate and recuperate. More terrible, you'll likewise take a chance with medical conditions and in any event, overtraining.

To cut after a building stage regardless have muscle to show for it, begin with a moderate shortfall of just 500 calories — it's the perfect number to start fat misfortune without forfeiting muscle size or strength gains. Keep tabs on your development like clockwork as muscle versus fat ratio, circuit estimations, and photographs to guarantee you're on the correct course.

Chapter Four

Demonstrated Ways to Lose Weight Without Working Out

1.   Eat Lots of Protein

Protein is a force to be reckoned with. In addition to the fact that it is fundamental for our wellbeing, however it can expand sensations of completion and diminish hunger. Along these lines, protein can assist you with eating less calories… and get thinner thus.

Investigations have discovered that rising protein from 15% to 30% assisted members with losing a normal of 11 pounds more than 12 weeks and eat 441 less calories every day, without purposefully limiting any food varieties or working out. So if you have any desire to shed pounds without practice or severe slimming down, begin by increasing your protein consumption. Have a go at having eggs for breakfast rather than breakfast oats, or add almonds over the course of the day as a tidbit.

2.   Hydrate

Remaining hydrated is critical to shedding pounds. Many individuals botch indications of drying out for hunger, and eat when they're parched as opposed to getting a beverage. At the point when you hydrate over the course of the day, you can keep away from drying out.

Drinking water, especially before a feast, can likewise assist you with eating less. At the point when you drink a huge glass of water prior to eating, you will commonly eat less calories. Assuming that you supplant sweet drinks with water, you will see significantly more noteworthy weight reduction.

## 3.	Keep Unhealthy Food Out of Reach

Can we just be real for a minute: for the majority of us, in the event that we have desserts, snacks, and other undesirable food around, it is hard to not eat it. That can be an issue on the off chance that we are attempting to get more fit. Yet, generally speaking, you want to keep these food varieties around for other relatives, visitors, or various different reasons.

One method for assisting you with keeping away from allurement is by reserving these food varieties out of your span. In the event that you keep chips and treats on the counter, you might go after those when you're ravenous or need a bite. Be that as it may, assuming you keep a bowl of natural product on the counter all things considered, you are bound to go with a better decision when you need to chomp on something.

4.   Eat Plenty of Fiber

Fiber is incredible for our bodies. Besides the fact that it diminishes the gamble of specific sorts of malignant growths, it can likewise assist with causing you to feel more full. That is on the grounds that thick fiber — the thoughtful found in plant-based food sources — structures a gel when it comes into contact with water. This gel builds the retention of supplements, and dials back how much time that it takes to purge your stomach.

So if you have any desire to get in shape, center around getting bunches of fiber in your eating routine. There are bunches of incredible high fiber choices, similar to beans, asparagus, oranges, and apples.

5.   Utilize Smaller Plates for Higher Calorie Foods

As of late, our plate sizes have developed altogether. At the point when we utilize enormous plates, it can make our piece sizes look a lot more modest than they really are — which might prompt weight gain. Paradoxically, when we utilize more modest plates, our segments look greater, which can trick our brains into imagining that we are eating more than we are.

Our cerebrums assume a significant part in weight reduction. On the off chance that you're hoping to shed a couple of pounds (or more), ponder how you plate your food. By picking dishes that are a lot more modest than normal, you might observe that you are happy with a more modest measure of food.

6.   Watch Your Portion Size

One of the main sources of weight gain in the United States is wild part estimates. Whenever we are served (or serve ourselves) large amounts of food, we are bound to eat beyond the place of completion. This can prompt weight gain and stoutness.

If you have any desire to get more fit without working out, just decreasing your part size can be a major assistance. Joined with eating gradually and drinking heaps of water, making this basic stride can permit you to diminish calories and drop weight.

7.   Be Mindful While Eating

In our furious lives, it is frequently enticing to perform various tasks. Maybe you're having lunch at your work area, or looking at your telephone while sitting in front of the TV. While completing a few things without a moment's delay can frequently bring about more prominent proficiency, on the off chance that you're occupied when you are eating, it can make you eat significantly an overabundance. Investigations have discovered that you will lose more weight when you practice careful eating.

Rather than eating on the sofa while sitting in front of the TV, while working, or while on your telephone, put away opportunity to eat without interruptions. Focus on your body and the signs that it is sending while you are eating.

This can assist you with eating significantly less nevertheless is full.

8.   Get Plenty of Sleep

An absence of rest can disturb the development of specific chemicals in our body that direct hunger. At the point when you don't get sufficient rest, or you get unfortunate rest, you might have expanded hunger and need undesirable, unhealthy food sources. Assuming that you are keen on shedding pounds, center around getting sufficient rest consistently. A decent night's rest will assist you with accomplishing your weight reduction objectives.

9.   Keep away from Sugar

It is absolutely impossible to get around it: sugar is scrumptious. However, when we consume an excess of sugar, it can adversely influence our wellbeing, making us put on weight and endangering us for various sicknesses, like diabetes.

At the point when we polish off sweet food varieties and beverages, it frequently doesn't encourage us. Accordingly, we might take in a lot more calories and put on weight. A genuinely straightforward method for getting in shape is to remove all sweet beverages, similar to pop and squeezes, and supplant them with water. You can likewise remove added sugars by restricting your sweet admission and picking lower sugar forms of your #1 food varieties.

10.   Have a go at Using Red Plates

This tip might sound peculiar, yet research has demonstrated the way that utilizing red plates can prompt diminished calorie consumption. While we don't know precisely why this procedure works, it appears to assist individuals with eating less unfortunate bites — maybe in light of the fact that we partner red with the word stop. Assuming that you have red plates at your home, think about plating fatty food sources on them, and see what occurs.

11.   Keep a Food Journal

Responsibility is an immense piece of any weight reduction venture. One method for staying responsible is to keep a diary of what you are eating, and when you are eating it. Along these lines, you can follow your food admission, and even note times when you are bound to tumble off of the so-called cart. You can involve pen and paper for a food diary, or any of various applications.

12.   Gauge Yourself Regularly

The most ideal way to be aware on the off chance that you're gaining ground with weight reduction — or falling away from the faith into weight gain — is to understand what you gauge. While gauging yourself again and again can be counterproductive (since your weight can vary over the course of the day), it is really smart to gauge yourself consistently so you know whether you are acquiring or getting thinner. You can remember your everyday load for your food diary.

In the event that you notice an addition, you can change your eating routine as needs be. On the off chance that you see a drop, you will be urged — and spurred to continue onward with your eating routine arrangement.

13.   Watch Snacking

We as a whole love having tidbits, whether we pack treats for an excursion, keep something reserved in our work area cabinet at work, or break out the popcorn while watching a film. The issue is that it tends to be difficult to monitor precisely the amount we are eating when we are nibbling.

Having sound snacks over the course of the day can assist with moving your digestion along. The key is to ensure that you are representing those bites — and monitoring the parts.

14. Keep away from Fad Diets

Assuming that you are hoping to get in shape, it tends to be difficult to keep away from the draw of an eating regimen that guarantees that you'll get more fit quick by drinking a couple of shakes a day, or only high temp water with some lemon, cayenne pepper, and maple syrup. While you might get in shape on these sorts of diets, it basically isn't reasonable.

Over the long haul, causing craze diets can harm your digestion. Accordingly, it'll be that a lot harder to get in shape over the long haul. Assuming that you are significant about weight reduction, stay away from juice purges, cabbage soup consumes fewer calories, and other undesirable eating regimens.

15.   Deal with Your Gut Health

The study of weight reduction is convoluted, and not completely perceived. In any case, scientists are starting to connect stoutness with an irregularity of particular kinds of microorganisms in our guts. You can resolve these issues by taking a day to day probity or eating matured food sources, the two of which can support your stomach wellbeing.

16.   Get Lots of Vitamin D

While researchers don't precisely comprehend the connection between Vitamin D and weight reduction, scientists have noticed that heavier individuals will generally have lower levels of vitamin D in their blood. At the point when individuals get more fit, they will generally encounter an expansion in vitamin D levels.

You can help your Vitamin D levels by taking an enhancement, getting more sun, or eating food varieties plentiful in Vitamin D. Doing so may assist you with shedding pounds, as well as getting added benefits like more grounded bones.

17.   Plan to Succeed

There is a familiar adage, "inability to plan is getting ready to fall flat." This is especially evident with regards to weight reduction.

Setting up your dinners ahead of time and ensuring that you have a lot of sound choices accessible can assist you with shedding pounds. At the point when you don't have great choices, you might be enticed to arrange a pizza or select up undesirable take food. By ensuring that you have simple dinners all set, you can keep away from these fatty snares and remain focused.

18.   Eat Good Fats

Before, fat got a terrible standing in the eating regimen local area. All the more as of late, researchers have found that particular sorts of fats are great for our bodies. These supposed great fats, similar to those tracked down in fish, nuts, avocados, and olive oil, can assist us with engrossing additional supplements from our food and even assist us with feeling more full for longer. By adding a moderate measure of solid fats to your eating regimen, you might have the option to lose more weight.

19.   Reconsider Your Morning Coffee

In a time where there is by all accounts a Starbucks everywhere, it is quite simple to accidentally consume 500 calories or more with your morning joe. In the event that you are prone to get a latte while heading to work, think about changing to some espresso (without added sugars) at home. Doing so could save you huge amount of cash and calories over the long run.

20.   Select Your Oils Carefully

Particular sorts of vegetable oil are known to be high in omega-6 unsaturated fats, which can make irritation and lead weight gain. Assuming you are hoping to get more fit, stay away from canola and soybean oil, and pick additional virgin olive oil all things being equal.

21.   Convey a Water Bottle Everywhere You Go

Above, we noticed that drinking heaps of water can assist you with getting thinner. One simple method for ensuring that you do this is by taking a water bottle with you as you approach your day. With bunches of extraordinary choices for sharp water bottles that save your refreshment cold for quite a long time, it is more straightforward than at any other time to ensure that you get enough H20. Furthermore, when you have a water bottle with you, you'll be bound to taste from it instead of getting a fatty espresso, pop, or other refreshment.

22.   Remember a Healthy Snack

We are in general occupied, and a significant number of us go through our days running starting with one thing then onto the next. At the point when you're making the rounds, sound bites and feasts aren't accessible 100% of the time. One method for keeping away from that particular situation is to convey a sound nibble with you. Keeping a bunch of almonds or a solid protein bar can assist you with trying not to pig out on more fatty quick food varieties or eatery feasts.

Chapter Five

Other Ways to Lose Weight Without Working Out

1.   Stock Your Freezer

We have all been in circumstances when we simply don't have the opportunity or energy to get to the store or to cook. For the majority of us, this might prompt requesting conveyance, which can be fine for a treat — yet not in the event that you are attempting to get more fit. All things being equal, ensure that your cooler is brimming with good feasts (like additional parts of soup), frozen veggies, and pre-divided protein. Like that, you'll have the option to eat on the table quick, without racing to the store or going through hours cooking.

2.   Make Healthy Foods the Star of Your Kitchen

Prior, we discussed how you ought to put undesirable food varieties, similar to desserts and pungent bites, in a harder-to-get to put in your kitchen to assist you with keeping away from enticement. The other side of this tip is that you ought to place quality food sources in simple to arrive at areas to make it almost certain that you will pick them all things considered.

Assuming you're attempting to eat all the more entire grains, for instance, it will be simpler to meet your objective if the quinoa and bulgar are at the front of your storage room, as opposed to covered toward the back. Put yourself in a good position by making it as simple as conceivable to get to quality food sources in your kitchen.

3.   Improve Your Food

The pattern of capturing your dinner for virtual entertainment can a piece disturb. However when you intend to snap a pic of something that you made, you are bound to stack it up with solid leafy foods. A delightfully pre-arranged feast is frequently viewed as seriously fulfilling, which can assist you with having lunch. So require a couple of additional minutes and make your food look phenomenal — then, at that point, snap a pic, and partake in the additional weight reduction reward.

4.   Slash Up Veggies for Easy Snacks or Meal Prep

At the point when you're occupied, it very well may be difficult to get thinner effectively in light of the fact that practicing good eating habits takes time. One strategy for getting around that is to continuously prepare sure that you have new veggies to eat or use in a recipe.

In the wake of purchasing vegetables at the market, wash and hack them once you return home. Like that, you can get some celery rather than pretzels, and you can have carrots prepared to throw into a recipe. Investing a touch of energy every week to make these strides can assist you with dropping load over the long run.

5.   Prepare Your Lunch

Eating out during your work day is in many cases a decent break, and a method for mingling. However eatery feasts are much of the time fatty, and stacked with undesirable fats. To manage your spending plan and your waistline, pack a solid lunch loaded up with great fats and veggies all things considered.

6.   Take a Lunch Break

Subsequent to preparing your lunch, consider adding another thing to your day to day daily practice — a touch of unwinding. Work can be unpleasant, and having lunch at your work area, or even in the workplace break room, doesn't permit you to get a psychological or actual break.

All things considered, track down a recreation area or green space close to your office. Take your lunch there, when weather conditions permits, and appreciate people watching, paying attention to music or a web recording, or just being without anyone else.

7.   Eliminate Food from Your Work Area

It is normal in numerous working environments to have snacks out, or a bowl of treats right in front of you.

However when these food varieties are promptly free, it improves the probability that you'll chow down on them — in any event, when you're not exactly ravenous. One method for combating this issue is to eliminate food from your visual perception at work. All things being equal, keep solid tidbits set aside in a work area cabinet or another area. No longer of any concern!

8.   Cut Your Alcohol Intake

A significant number of us partake in a glass of wine, a lager, or a blended beverage toward the finish of a drawn out day. While savoring liquor control can be sound (especially red wine), it can likewise prompt weight gain. Liquor doesn't give sustenance, yet it tends to be high in calories. By disposing of or lessening your liquor admission, you can cut calories and get in shape.

9.   Select Your Sides Carefully

Eating out can be a minefield. Indeed, even apparently solid dishes, similar to veggies, are much of the time doused in spread and salt. Regardless of whether you request a good dinner, it might accompany an unhealthy side. Get into the act of continuously requesting a serving of mixed greens as your side — instead of fries, pureed potatoes, or some other undesirable choice. Along these lines, you can in any case partake in your primary dish, while cutting calories simultaneously.

10.   Request Half to Go

This is an old stunt, however a decent one while eating out at an eatery. Segment sizes at eateries are crazy — and not right at the Cheesecake Factory (which is notable for its monstrous, excessively full plates of food). If you have any desire to partake in a dinner out without being enticed to clean your plate, address the issue head on: request half of your feast to be boxed up to go, so it is never at any point on the table.

11.   Try not to Let Others Serve You

At the point when another person makes a plate for you, or cuts you a piece of cake, they may not be mindful so as to guarantee that you are getting a fitting part. You can abstain from indulging at social occasions by serving yourself. Like that, you can ensure that you are getting a plate that has a perfect proportion of food.

12.   Investigate New Recipes

It is not difficult to get into a trench with cooking, and to depend on recipes that are soothing or nostalgic. While it isn't awful to enjoy solace food sources like macaroni and cheddar infrequently, it can keep you from investigating a novel, new thing — and better. Invest some energy riding the web or going through cookbooks for present day, good dinners to attempt.

13.   Be Wary of "Diet" Foods

A ton of food sources are named "diet," offering seemingly a simple method for cutting calories. Be that as it may, But a great deal of these food varieties are stacked with counterfeit sugars, similar to consume less calories pop, which can really make you desire desserts — despite the fact that the sugars contain no genuine sugar. By keeping away from diet food varieties and adhering to genuine, entire food varieties, you might have the option to cut calories.

14.   Attempt an Elimination Diet

Many individuals are delicate to particular sorts of food, similar to gluten or dairy. On the off chance that you truly do have a food prejudice or sensitivity, it can prompt swelling, distress, and even weight gain. In the event that you feel awkward subsequent to eating a specific food, consider going on an end diet. You might find that by removing particular sorts of food, you feel significantly improved — and even drop pounds.

15.   Adhere to a Routine

There is a well-known axiom: "in the event that it ain't down and out, don't fix it." When it comes to consuming less calories, it is completely fine to adhere to what you know. This might mean making seven days of dinners on Sunday, or having similar breakfast and snacks consistently. At the point when you have a cooler brimming with food that you realize that you can eat, it decreases the probability of you going for a comfort thing that isn't as sound.

16.   Invest Energy Outdoors

Stress can prompt weight gain. Assuming you think of yourself as wrecked, feeling blue, or recently exhausted, getting outside can assist you with getting some alleviation. You can go for a climb or a walk, or just invest energy in a recreation area. The significant thing is simply being in nature, which can work on your emotional wellness and mind-set.

17.   Keep away from Family Style Meals

A considerable lot of us grew up eating family style, with all of the supper choices on the table, so everybody can serve themselves. While putting all that on the table is more helpful than dishing up individual plates in the kitchen, it can make it simpler to gorge. On the off chance that you need to get up and stroll to the kitchen to get a subsequent serving, you might mull over whether you are truly ravenous.

18.   Simply Say No to the Bread Basket

At the point when you eat out in a café, the server frequently brings a bushel of rolls or chips and salsa. It very well may be hard to not dive in, particularly assuming that you come into the eatery hungry. Be that as it may, these kinds of free starters are normally fatty and filling. All things considered, have a little protein-finished nibble prior to making a beeline for eat — or request a verdant green serving of mixed greens to begin.

19.   Turn Down the Heat

As we head into winter, this might seem like an odd tip when you maintain that your home should be warm and comfortable. Yet, keeping your home just somewhat cooler can assist you with getting thinner. Why? Since when your body is cool, it needs to work harder to remain warm — which can assist you with getting more fit.

20.   Attempt Nuts As a Healthy Snack

Incidentally, squirrels have the right thought. Nuts are an extraordinary food, loaded up with protein, solid fats, and fiber, all of which assists you with remaining full longer. Simply ensure that you monitor the number of nuts you're that eating, as they will generally be higher in calories.

21.   Get the Day Going Right

At the point when you get up toward the beginning of the day, your body has been fasting for 8-12 hours or significantly longer. You might be enticed to have a little breakfast on the off chance that you're attempting to get more fit. Incidentally, doing so can really misfire. All things being equal, have a go at having a major breakfast — in a perfect world highlighting eggs as a decent wellspring of protein. Having a greater breakfast can really assist you with eating less during the day, which means weight reduction.

22.   Try not to Skip Breakfast

You might feel that skirting a dinner will assist you with shedding pounds. Assuming you're behind schedule in the first part of the day, or simply could do without breakfast food sources, you might be enticed to skip breakfast... however you ought to try not to do that. At the point when you don't have breakfast, you are probably going to eat more all through the remainder of the day — including a major supper, which can make you put on weight. Eat a sound, filling breakfast consistently to help your weight reduction.

23.   Consider What Goes on Your Plate

Numerous Americans are utilized to an eating routine that is weighty on meat and carbs, and light on products of the soil. To get in shape, change everything around.

Envision your plate as being parted into thirds. Top off 66% of your plate with lean protein and vegetables, then the leftover third with entire grains.

24.   Drink Tea

Tea might be less famous than espresso in the United States, yet you shouldn't neglect this nourishing force to be reckoned with. A few kinds of tea, including cinnamon and mint tea, can really assist you with shedding pounds. Mint is a craving suppressant, while cinnamon can diminish glucose levels. Peppermint tea may likewise assist your body with processing fats. Simply avoid sugar while going with your drink of decision.

25.   Make Losing Weight Easy With Smart Swaps

There are not many things that are superior to a major plate of pasta. However customary spaghetti and different types of pasta are loaded with calories. Rather than pasta, attempt a solid other option, similar to spaghetti squash or zucchini noodles. Not exclusively will you cut calories with these savvy trades, you'll likewise support your veggie admission.

26.   Attempt a Squirt of Lemon

Ideally, you're drinking a ton of water over the course of the day to remain hydrated. To support your weight reduction, take a stab at adding a lemon to your water. Lemons have various supplements that can really diminish pressure and lift weight reduction, including Vitamin C, polyphenols, and gelatin. It likewise assists with extinguishing your thirst and adds a pleasant flavor to your beverage!

27.   Nibble Brilliantly

Nibbling can be a significant method for firing up your digestion — on the off chance that you eat the ideal things with flawless timing. In a perfect world, save your snacks for mid-evening to fuel your weight reduction. Studies have shown that individuals who nibble in the first part of the day, as opposed to the evening, will generally eat more throughout the day.

Chapter Six

Eat Healthy Live Healthy

1.   Try not to Drink Your Calories

Getting a soft drink around mid-afternoon, a lager around evening time, or savoring juice the morning might appear to be sufficiently blameless. However these beverages all have a ton of calories — and won't top you off. Rather than drinking your calories, gobble something beneficial to top you off and give you energy.

2.   Pause and Think

Large numbers of us who battle with our weight do so in light of the fact that we eat when we aren't really eager. We might eat down potato chips when we are exhausted, search out frozen yogurt when we are miserable, or stop at a drive-through following an unpleasant day at work. While this is a typical survival strategy, it's anything but a solid one. So before you eat, require a moment to check in with yourself. Sort out whether or not you're truly eager, or on the other hand in the event that you are attempting to deal with your feelings with food.

3.   Become Smart about Nutrition

Food is fuel for our bodies, yet not many of us really figure out nourishment. Fortunately you don't need to go to class to find out about what is best for your body. Perusing names is a decent beginning, however you can accomplish something significantly easier: pay attention to your body. Scarfing down a small bunch of sticky bears during a midday rut might give you a brief lift, yet how does your body feel a short time later? Contemplate what encourages you, and go from that point.

4.   Attempt Meal Prepping

Setting up a lot of feasts early may not appear to be energizing. In any case, having pre-distributed dinners all set can assist you with remaining focused with your eating regimen, and make it simple for you to pursue solid decisions. Invest some energy exploring recipes, and afterward commit a couple of hours every week to ensuring that you have a scope of choices all set.

5.   Establish a Soothing Environment for Meal Times

Studies have shown that when you eat some place that is brilliant and uproarious, you will generally eat more.

Diminishing the lights and bringing down the commotion can really assist you with eating less by decreasing the probability that you will race through your dinner.

6.   Converse with Your Doctor About Weight Gain

At times, weight gain might be connected with an ailment. In the event that you have unexplained weight gain or really can't get in shape, it could be the ideal opportunity for an examination or a physical. You might have a hidden condition that has made you placed on pounds or made it hard for you to drop weight.

7.   Track Calories With A Weight Loss App

Counting calories might appear to be dreary and outdated, however it tends to be an effective method for ensuring that you're not eating excessively. It is likewise a lot more straightforward than any time in recent memory, with a scope of calorie following applications accessible. Pick one that addresses your issues, and get to following!

Getting thinner can be amazingly troublesome. For the typical American, adhering to a severe eating routine and exercise system is almost difficult to do while adjusting the requests of work and family. Also, abstaining from excessive food intake and exercise may not actually work whenever done mistakenly. Luckily, there is a superior method for losing a groundbreaking measure of weight without extreme actual work.

Weight reduction without practice is conceivable. Ideal You offers precisely exact thing you really want to lose a groundbreaking measure of weight rapidly while never swinging by a rec center. Our weight reduction plan offers all-normal food-based supplements, customary gatherings with weight reduction mentors, an organized food list and a weight reduction diary. Our emphasis is on rebalancing your body to reset your digestion. We give you the training and devices you want to get more fit in a solid, maintainable way.

Conclusion

Any individual who has attempted to get in shape knows exactly the way in which hard it very well may be. While it very well may be genuinely simple to pack on pounds, dropping them can be amazingly troublesome.

Individuals frequently prescribe practice as a method for getting thinner. While there are various medical advantages to resolving, standard activity will not be guaranteed to assist you with thinning down. That is on the grounds that exercise never really changes the hormonal uneven characters that frequently fuel weight gain - and make it hard to get in shape.

Assuming you're hoping to get more fit without working out, you have come to the ideal locations. Ideal you offers a protected, powerful method for getting more fit without dialing back your digestion or making you go through tiresome exercises. We'll tell you the very best way to shed pounds without working out. Beneath, we have illustrated probably the best ways to get thinner while never going to an exercise center. Altogether, there are more than 60 unique ways of getting in shape without working out.